DETOX
YOUR SOUL

RENOVATE YOUR MIND, BODY AND SPIRIT

Tamar House

Detox Your Soul

Copyright © 2013 by Tamar House

ISBN 978-1-62847-424-4

This book is dedicated to my parents, my husband and my children. They love me from the "grass to God's house"!

A NOTE FROM THE AUTHOR

When I was growing up, my father, a therapist, would always encourage me to talk about my feelings. Instead of getting upset at me, he would insist on talking to me about what I'd done wrong. As a teenager, I hated this more than anything. I'd rather get yelled at or have my pager taken away than *talk*.

It was so hard discussing my feelings, but I had no choice. Those were the rules. My mother was pretty easy going, but very structured. She kept a very clean and neat home, and everything had its place at all times. She was very introverted, so she didn't talk much at all. She was so shy that she'd even have me return items to the store for her so she didn't have to talk to the clerks.

Because I was forced to talk early on, I talked to everyone. I was taught to stand up for what was right and admit when I was wrong. Then I was told that my father was not my biological father. I started feeling that I wasn't good enough and lost my voice for a few years.

In junior high, I went to a private Christian school that didn't believe in dancing. I didn't understand. The Bible said it was good to dance. Ecclesiastes 3:4 states, there is "a time to weep, and a time to laugh; a time to mourn and a time to dance". I was sure that we were supposed to celebrate life by dancing, so I fought this with the board of directors at the school.

I was shot down, but my teacher, Miss Cindy Dodd, fought with me, believed with me, and celebrated with me by allowing us to have a dance at her house!

At that special event, I realized that I had to stand up for what I believed in to help others who did not have the courage to do the same. I also learned early on that I might not get what I expected in return, but that, in time, God would reward me for my actions some-how, some way.

This learned behavior allowed me to realize my voice. It felt good to have such encouragement from my friends. The support was amaz-ing! I still wondered why my biological father left my mother before I was even born, but I kept that buried deep down.

Even though I'd grown up in a Protestant church, I attended a Catholic high school, where I often argued with the religion teach-ers—not out of disrespect, but out of curiosity about how two religions that believed in the same God could be so different.

I was often sent to the Dean's office, but when I recited the Bible verse that supported my actions, they always let me go back to class.

I spent most of my teenage years getting into trouble… mostly because I wanted to push my limits to see who would stand up for the truth. I was rebellious and tested my parents often. (Sorry, Mom and Dad! I love you with all my heart, and I truly apologize for all that I put you through.) But I also had learned who my biological father was and tested the waters with kids that I met who were really my cous-ins. I thought by acting out, my father would come to rescue me. Not the case. He never came, and I grew more distant from my parents and rebelled even more.

I got married at an early age to a man that I knew wasn't good for me. I so desperately wanted a family of my own, that I overlooked what was best for me, choosing to follow my heart and not my head. I somehow lost my voice during my marriage, but, after meeting with a therapist and realizing that our marriage would never work, I found the courage deep inside me again.

When I looked at my beautiful son and realized that it's better to be *from* a broken home than to be *in* one, I found my voice again. I packed up my clothes and the baby and left for good.

For the next few years, I felt free and ready to conquer the world! I partied a lot and strayed from God. It felt good at the time, but I then began dating a man that I thought would "rescue" me. Not only did he *not* rescue me, he also left me while I was pregnant. The stress from that sent me to the hospital for months with pre-term labor. During the two months I spent in the hospital, I had a lot of time to think about my life and my decisions.

After my second son was born on Valentine's Day, 2003, I decided that I would only allow positive thoughts to control my life.

I realized my failure to rid my life of negative thoughts and people was what had caused me to become involved in bad relationships. Because I allowed myself to listen to that negative voice inside my head, I suffered for years. My family suffered for years. My kids suffered for years.

After spending a few years in therapy, I finally figured out what I was doing wrong: I was thinking wrong, hanging around the wrong people, doing the wrong things. I strayed far from God. It was time to detox my soul. So I did!

I got rid of a few bad habits, a few so-called friends, and even a few toxic family members. I finally had room in my heart for the positive things God had in store for me all along. I softened my heart and prepared myself for the man God wanted me to find.

In 2010, I met the man of my dreams. Ryan and I have now been happily married for a few years. We have four beautiful children and reside in Valencia, California. We both are strong Christians and belong to Real Life Church. We both have successful careers in real estate. He's in commercial office leasing and sales, and I do residential sales and leasing. He helped me find the courage to finally confront my biological father, who basically said that he wanted nothing to do with me now or then. I was thankful that I was able to put that behind me. Good or bad, it was a finite answer. This was the one final thing in my life for which I needed closure. It was scary and strange, but I did it. I was finally able to move forward and completely detox my soul. I realized that I, and I alone, am in charge of my thoughts. And it feels great!

I hope you enjoy reading this book as much as I enjoyed writing it. You should be proud of yourself for taking this first step to *Detox Your Soul*! Enjoy! God Bless!

CONTENTS

INTRODUCTION

*W*hat is happiness, and how do we find it in today's busy society? That seems to be the question on the minds of so many people.

Life has become a juggling act: men and women everywhere are trying to balance the demands of their jobs, homes, and families. Our economy has pushed people into working longer hours to make ends meet.

Our children are over-scheduled with activities to keep them active. Between our jobs and shuffling our children from activity to activity, we leave little to no time for our own mental and physical nourishment.

We have become a society of people hooked on technology. Television and video games have become our outlet for the few snippets of downtime that we can muster. In a nutshell, many of us are feeling exhausted and powerless to change our endless cycle of depression and unhappiness.

This book is about recreating your habits and defining a fulfilling life. The happier you are as an individual, the happier everyone around you will be. This process starts with re-engineering a new you.

Back in the 1970s, author Max Malt wrote a book called *Psycho-Cybernetics*, the premise of which was that any habit could be broken in 21 days. Designing your own life is as simple as breaking your old, unhealthy habits and developing new, healthier ways of living. There is a catch to all of this "habit-breaking" though; you have to *want* to make your life better.

Habits are easier to make than they are to break. If you repeat a behavior often enough, your synaptic nerve pathways are going to get worn in. The human brain is an adaptive piece of machinery.

Can you really break a habit in 21 days?

Every mind works in different ways. In order to break a habit, you first have to be conscious that the habit exists. Based on my experience, anyone who is aware of a habit and is motivated enough to break it, can. Like anything in life, breaking habits requires practice to develop mastery.

If you have purchased this book, you may be ready to commit to making your life more manageable. This book will help you identify the areas in your life that need to be cleared out and re-organized to make room for the new, healthy habits you desire. This book will also guide you through a twenty-one day transformation, and provide you with the support you need after you shift your consciousness to becoming the person you've always known you could become.

Congratulations! Today may be the first day of the rest of your wonderful life!

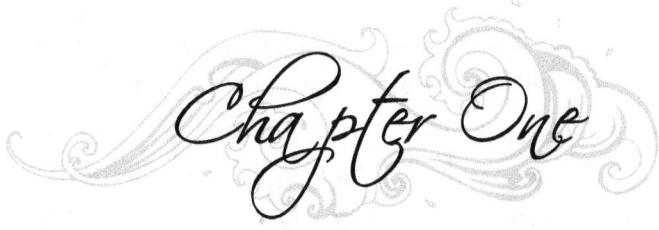

THE BALANCING ACT

*D*etoxing your soul may sound like a tall order, so we will start at the beginning.

The first step in bringing your life into focus is finding balance. Now, you are probably thinking "how?" The best way is to evaluate which parts of your life are out of balance.

Many people juggle the demands of their jobs and the rest of their lives, so you are not alone. You can take some small steps right away to free up time.

Many people put in extra hours at work, because they feel overwhelmed. Do you really *need* to put in extra hours, or can you manage your work time more efficiently?

Let's work smarter, not harder.

At work, many people spend time socializing. I remember a job where everyone stood around and drank coffee and gossiped for the first thirty minutes every morning. Since I did not drink coffee, I used to go straight to my desk and start work.

At the end of the day, I would get ready to leave and my supervisor would mention that it would be nice if I could stay and help out some of my co-workers.

I was not very popular when I suggested that my co-workers would be more productive if they cut out the chitchat every morning.

After my supervisor made it clear that this was a "teamwork" position, I began to look for a new job. I wasn't opposed to being a team player—I was opposed to picking up the slack of others who spent their work time frivolously, and giving up time with my family to do so.

Technology can also be a time-waster at work. Most of us have smart phones that are supposed to streamline our lives, but they can turn into time-wasters if you spend your work time texting, Facebooking, Tweeting, and playing video games.

Set clear boundaries with yourself about how much time you spend on the phone; for example, only pick up your phone between certain pre-set hours. You can even set your voicemail to reflect those hours and set expectations for your clients.

Outside of work, manage your time better by getting rid of draining activities. Many people waste time on activities that add no value to their lives. Interacting with friends is nice, but what about that friend that complains all the time or spends hours talking about the boyfriend who won't commit? Listening is a great quality to have, but don't waste your time on people who are "stuck" in their own lives.

You might be asking, "How do I know if someone is stuck?" Do you keep having the same conversation with someone over and over? Does the person you spend time with always talk about the same topic? It's one thing to talk about your common interests, but, if your friend talks or complains continuously about the same topic with no resolution to the problem, they may be stuck.

What about your time on the Internet? Have you ever sat down to look something up and realized that you are still on the same website an hour later? It's easy to get caught up chatting with a friend or reading posts, but it's time to minimize those activities.

If you must engage in these activities daily, set reasonable time limits and stick to them.

Another way to free up more time is to outsource your errands and household chores. Could you order your groceries online and have them delivered? Would it be cost-effective to hire a neighbor kid to mow your lawn?

Is there a dry cleaner in your neighborhood that will pick up and deliver? Even if you are on a budget, you may find the time you gain to be worth a little extra expense.

You may have other friends who are willing to help out. Carpooling with the kids to school or extra-curricular activities will help alleviate some of the stress in your life.

Make time to exercise. You are probably thinking, "Yeah right, I don't have time," but exercise may help you get more done by increasing your focus and energy levels.

Research has shown that exercise helps people become more alert. Try fitting in a thirty-minute walk on your lunch hour.

What about that time that you spend driving back and forth from your children's activities? Can you park and walk while they are at piano lessons or playing soccer, instead of socializing with the other parents that are standing around watching? You might even find that a parent or two would like to join you.

Learning to relax will also help you manage your time more efficiently. Take twenty minutes a day and completely decompress. Enjoy a bubble bath, take a walk, listen to music, or learn to meditate. Do something that will soothe your soul. "Me time" is so important to our well-being, and, yet, so many people are busy nurturing everyone else around them, they forget about themselves.

You don't have to jump into "me time" with both feet. Start small with twenty minutes a day. Slowly add activities into your schedule that are important to you.

Leave the office early one day a week; plan a relaxing getaway once a year, or budget an hour a week on a new hobby.

If you are married, make sure that your spouse does the same. You will both be more refreshed and ready to embrace your family time together.

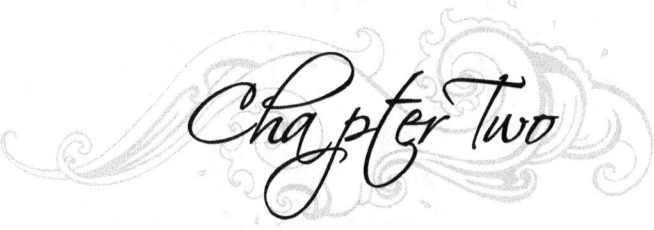

BE REAL OR BE MISERABLE

*B*efore you can start analyzing, you need to think about how you are going to be authentic in this process and in your life.

What does it mean to live in authentic connection?

Authenticity is the permission we give ourselves to be real. This means to be who we are, consciously aware of our good points, and our points that are not so great.

Authenticity is when we consciously love others, our lives, and ourselves whole-heartedly.

Being authentic means that we have the courage to face our fears. This does not mean things like your fear of spiders, but the fears that you have surrounding intimacy, connection, and relationships. These fears are existential fears such as being rejected, abandoned, or judged as not good enough. We cannot eliminate these fears; they are present to teach us, allow us to grow, and transform our relationships.

At its root, fear of intimacy is the fear of knowing ourselves up close and personal. We all fear that we will not like what we see if we closely examine our inner beings.

Analyzing your journal, for example, is not about eliminating your weaknesses; it is about embracing them, accepting them, and loving them. To love yourself and others is an act of audacity. Once you are able to accept yourself, accepting others becomes second nature.

Acting authentically is about challenging memories that we all carry, and redefining them. In some cases, it may mean that we take responsibility for actions that we have blamed on others. In other cases, acting authentically may mean letting go and forgiving others for events that have damaged us. When we are able to do this, we will find peace, harmony, and balance.

One of the points of analyzing this journal authentically is that you get to know yourself inside and out. This involves setting intentions, building awareness, and becoming conscious about who you are. As we will discuss in later chapters, it may mean confronting your inner child or setting an intention to lose weight. The goal is to understand how you acquired these bad habits, how to break them, and how to replace them with healthy ones.

Being authentic also means that you learn to accept yourself. All your flaws, mistakes, and successes *create* who you are. Accept that. They all belong to you. Once you begin to accept who you really are and become the real you instead of who other people want you to be, you will experience the freedom you have spent your whole life trying to find.

Unconditional love for oneself is also a part of acting authentically. Most people think that loving yourself means being selfish. This is a complete misconception. Loving yourself unconditionally means that you do what is best for you at all times. If something in your life feels uncomfortable, you speak up without fear and address the issue. You are bold and courageous in your expressions, regardless of what others think or try to push on you. You live by your own values and demand the respect you deserve.

Living with unconditional love for yourself will allow you to love those around you unconditionally as well. You will respect the boundaries of others because you act respectfully toward yourself. Living authentically means that you make choices with your heart and not just your head. You do not over-analyze situations, because you know what feels good and what does not. You will stop allowing others' opinions of what's best for you get in the way.

Learning to live in authenticity also means that you will start to recognize authenticity in others. The best example of this is in small children. Observe a child and watch how he or she lives in the moment. When children get angry, they express anger. There is never a fear that the people around them will not love them if they express anger openly.

Hiding our anger out of fear is something we are conditioned to do as we grow older. This may come in many forms. For example, a woman who doesn't express her anger and resentment over being ignored by her husband because she fears he may leave her.

Does authenticity mean that you throw a temper tantrum when you don't get your way? No, it simply means that you communicate how you feel in a calm manner, and then remove yourself from the situation. Don't expect the other person to change. Live in the moment, and know that you can't change anyone but yourself.

Recognizing people around you who are living authentically will help you start to make healthy friendships and realize which ones need to end. You may be confused at this point about what gets in the way of being authentic.

Probably the biggest issue is fear of what others think about you. Many of us spend our life thinking that the opinions of others matter more than those we have of ourselves. Many women take this on in the form of "people pleasing". Who didn't grow up with a mother who reminded you to change your underwear in case you got in an accident? *Really, Mom, if I am wearing dirty underwear, is it a reflection of your mothering skills?* Laughable when you think about it now!

You can identify this fear by assessing what behaviors you engage in to keep the peace, or so that others will accept you. When you are engaging in these activities, you are draining your own energy and not leaving space for new energy to come in. A good rule to follow is that, when a relationship no longer serves you and the other person, you go your separate ways. This is an essential step in making room for new people and new adventures. Sometimes, a friendship ends for no reason. There was no fight, nothing was done wrong. You both just stopped being friends. I have learned that friends come and go, and, still, your life goes on. You will make new friends. Every person that is in your life is there for a reason, a season, or a lifetime. When someone is in your life for a reason, it is usually because you have a need that they can meet. They may help you through a difficult time or provide guidance and support. They usually feel like your "guardian angel", and most of the time they are! The relationship usually ends rather quickly, and this is when you need to realize your desire has been fulfilled, and their work is done. Your prayer has been answered and it is now time to move on. Then there are those that are in your life for a season. A season of growth. This person will help you experience joy you have never imagined! Believe it! It's real! But it's only for a season. Lastly, there is the lifetime relationship. This relationship will teach lifetime lessons that will help you build a solid emotional foundation. Your job is to accept that person no matter what and love them unconditionally. That is what God has called each of us to do. Whether someone is in your life for a reason, a season, or a lifetime, be authentic.

Another way that we lose our authenticity is when we are trapped by the expectations of others. This happens frequently in family relationships or at work. We start to believe the stories around those expectations.

To give you an example: growing up, my friend's father frequently told her that she lacked common sense. When she would not do something the way he wanted it done, he would reiterate this statement to her.

As we grew up, she began to believe that she lacked common sense. Only later in life did she realize that she had a tremendous amount of common sense. Her father thought that his way of doing things was the "right" way, when there were many ways to accomplish the same tasks.

Watching my friend grow up with this poor self-worth made me careful not to repeat the same mistake with my children. When I give them a task, I let them figure out their own way of doing things. Sometimes I have to shake my head and laugh at the way they finish a task, but I do not criticize them about the way they accomplish it.

Sometimes, it's tough not to tell your children how to do things the "easier" way, as we usually know what gets the job done faster and with less stress. Allowing them to at least try it their way for a while, as long as they get the job done, increases their confidence.

At some point showing them how doing things "differently" may cause them less stress or save time, but "telling" them to do it "your way" may cause frustration for you both.

One pitfall of trying to behave authentically is going too far in the other direction. Do not let stubbornness get in the way of being authentic. If you have been a people-pleaser, you shouldn't suddenly become so selfish that you refuse to do anything for others.

It can be useful to swing in the other direction for the short term, while you experiment with boundaries; just be careful not to replace one negative habit with another.

As you become more authentic, you will also become more adept at identifying manipulation. Manipulation is what people who are not authentic do in order to get their way. By maintaining your authenticity, you stay true to your own needs and won't succumb to the manipulations of others.

Recognize manipulation as the other person's attempt to get what he or she wants from you without having to make changes in his or her own life.

Keep all of this in mind when you look back over the entries in your journal. Start to realize these issues in your current relationships. Is there someone who manipulates you? Have you tried talking to them? Has there been any change? If not, you may need to re-evaluate this relationship.

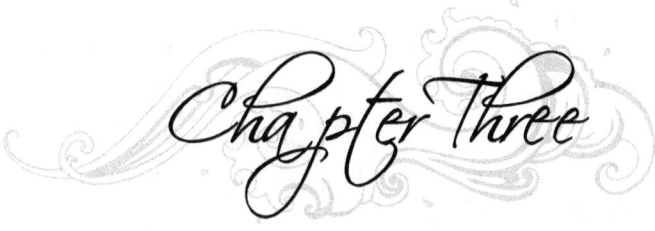

PREPARING FOR GREATNESS

Once you have made the decision that detoxing your soul leads you to find true happiness, it is time to make the necessary preparations. In order to change patterns in your life, you must become aware of them. Spending time alone with God will help you see your goals more clearly. Pray about this. Journaling will also help you accomplish the task of becoming aware. Change is a process, and it doesn't happen overnight. If change were easy, everyone would be doing it!

In this stage, you are motivated to uncover the patterns that hold you back from experiencing the life you crave. You are enthusiastic about your desire to become a better person, but what are the obstacles you face? You must be ready to take a leap of faith. Before you quit drinking or even start a new exercise program, you need to make preparations to really figure out why and how you are going to accomplish these new feats. Making changes without preparation may cause more stress, anxiety, frustration, and possibly contribute to failure.

Planning a life change is a lot like planning a vacation, only much more is at stake. Step one in this process is purchasing a notebook that you can use as a journal. Time to take inventory of your life. Carry this journal with you everywhere for the next week. You never know when an idea or piece of information will come to you that will be important for establishing a game plan for your future.

After you purchase the journal, write down the items you need to look at. Be one hundred percent truthful with your answers and observations. Write down the first things that come to your mind, and analyze your thoughts and feelings. Some of these areas are thought provoking and may surprise you.

During this process of analysis, be gentle with yourself. This means analyzing without judgment or guilt. Some of the areas of which you take stock may make you sad or angry. Take notice of these emotions and write them down. These are areas in your life where people, situations, and childhood emotions may be triggering patterned behavior. Recognizing these areas is important to your freedom.

Remember that the point of journaling is personal growth and development. By regularly recording your thoughts, you will gain insight into your behaviors. It has been proven that journaling used for problem-solving and stress reduction can improve your mental and physical health. We all have dark moods, bad days, and anxious feelings. Use journal writing to explore that darkness, and you will find your inner light.

The hardest part of journaling is just beginning. Here are some tips to get you started:

1. **Start writing about where you are in your life at this moment in time**. Don't worry about where you have been or where you are going. Start your journal in the present. There is a list of questions later in this chapter to help you begin your process.

2. **Set a timer for ten minutes to set your stream of consciousness**. This means that you write whatever comes to mind. No holding back or thinking about what you are writing and why—just ten minutes of free flow.

3. **If you are having a hard time writing, cut out magazine pictures that describe what you are thinking**. Make a visual picture to help you start writing; consider it a self-portrait.

4. **Cultivate an attitude of gratitude by writing things that are uplifting**. Perhaps you were inspired to gratitude by quotations or events. If you are having a hard time getting into a grateful place, take a few minutes outside and write about nature. The world we live in is a magical place. Start recording the things you notice: the sky, flowers, seasons, and anything else.

5. **If you are doing inner child work, write your dialogue with alternating hands**. An "inner child" can be defined as a person's supposed original or true self, especially when regarded as damaged or concealed by negative childhood experiences. Use your subdominant hand to represent questions or statements that your inner child has. Write answers with your dominant hand that you have now as an adult.

6. **Maintain a log of your successes**. Begin with some of your big successes and start adding small daily successes. You will quickly notice that you have small successes every day. Be proud.

7. **If you are struggling or disturbed by something, write about it in third person**. Writing in third person means writing as a person on the outside looking in—someone with no personal stake in the issue. This will give you distance and provide new

perspective. After writing in third person, read over your pages, and write down what you have learned about yourself.

8. **Learning to re-trust yourself.** Write down questions or concerns. Take a deep breath, and listen for a response from your Higher Self. Write down the response. If you do not get an answer right away, look for signs during the day. So many times, we are so busy that we do not take the time to stop and listen to what our intuition is trying to tell us. You will be relearning the value and joy of your wisdom. You will also take pride in making decisions without second-guessing yourself.

Here are some questions you need to answer honestly in your journal:

1. Who are the negative people in my life?
2. What are the bad foods I consume?
3. What causes me stress at home?
4. What causes me stress at work?
5. What makes my home life unbalanced?
6. What makes my work life unbalanced?
7. What makes my personal life unbalanced?
8. What do I do for exercise?
9. What do I do for "me time"?
10. What do I overindulge in?
11. What am I addicted to?
12. Do I have behaviors that I know are unhealthy?
13. What makes me angry?
14. What in my life makes me feel powerless?
15. How do I react when I am overwhelmed?

Review this list and your responses over the next few days. You may find that you start adding to the list as events throughout your day trigger responses. This may be an uncomfortable process—possibly very uncomfortable—but you need to be willing to get comfortable with being uncomfortable in order to make the changes necessary to achieve the life you *really* want.

Keep in mind that change is a difficult process and something that cannot be achieved overnight. Try not to be hard on yourself if change doesn't come as rapidly as you would like. Praise God for the work you have done so far, and celebrate! If you begin to feel overwhelmed, step back and take a break to get your bearings and add a new dimension of perspective.

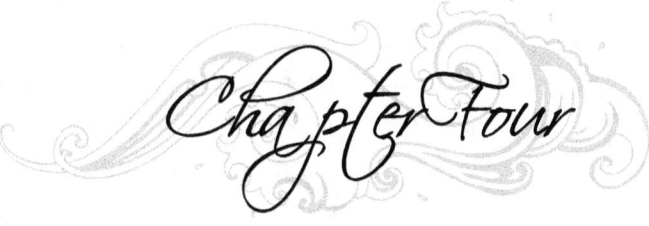

ME, ANALYZED

*I*t may have been weeks or months since you last picked up this book or your journal, but, regardless of how long it took you to get to this stage, give yourself a great big pat on the back. You were able to look yourself in the mirror, be honest with yourself, and confront what needed to be altered in your life. Now, it's time to analyze your journal results.

Take a look at what you've written down for each answer to the questions asked in the last chapter. Start a new page in your journal, and write down your thoughts to each of the questions. Make a chart of "good habits", "bad habits", and "new habits". Now you will become aware of which ones you need to nourish, which ones you need to expel, and which ones you need to create.

Chances are, you have been aware of some of your old "bad" habits for a while and have tried to break them before. Now is the time to write down what you have tried in the past. Take a hard look at the items in this part of the exercise. Can you identify why these past efforts didn't work? Write down honest answers to why they didn't work. Do you see a pattern? Do you self-sabotage? Did you really make an effort, or was it all sort of half-hearted? Did someone else sabotage your efforts?

What has worked in the past but didn't last? Write all of this down too. Was there a time issue? A discipline issue? Take a moment and write down the craziest thing you can think of to bring about the change you need. Alternately, write down the opposite of what you might do to bring about the change you want. Consider whether there is any validity to these options.

Once you have brainstormed the options to change your behavior, develop a list of the resources, which will help you as you create a plan to move forward. For instance, if you don't ever have the time to get out of the house to do something for yourself, write down some creative ways to start working towards accomplishing down time. Some suggestions:

Make a pact with your spouse to trade daily down time. A couple days a week, he goes to the gym after work, and on alternating days you take a yoga class while he cooks dinner and watches the kids.

Trade with a group of friends. "I will take your kids for a couple hours on Tuesdays, if you take mine for a couple hours on Thursdays."

Get help from parents or siblings. Simply plan a schedule at the start of every week so that everyone gets his or her own "me-time."

If you have children, and you want to spend your down time exercising, find a gym with childcare. Many gyms offer this as a perk.

Hire a housekeeper. Have someone come in and do the heavy housework once a week, so you can keep up the light, day-to-day work.

Organize the free time you have differently. For instance, when you arrive at a meeting early, you could return phone calls from the car, so you do not have to later. Read your e-mails and answer them if you are waiting in line at the grocery store. In other words, take small blocks of time that you would normally waste and make them productive.

Take twenty minutes when you get home from work and just meditate. Close the bedroom door, and lie down on the bed. Clear your head of all of the day's pressures. You will enter your family time refreshed and ready to leave work at the workplace.

Keep all of your options open when analyzing your journal entries. It also helps to make a "bucket list." Detail all of the things you would like to accomplish in the next couple of years. They don't have to be accomplished immediately, but keeping a list or making a dream board will help you focus on the things you want to do and get your mind thinking about methods to attain those goals.

Be sure you include items on that list that you can accomplish on your own. Not everything on that list has to benefit your spouse or your children. The fact that you accomplish tasks and goals on your own will only benefit everyone else in your life when you project a more positive self.

Keep all of the numbers and options handy as you enter the next phase, where you take action.

Lastly, analyze your inner chatter. Inner chatter is that voice inside your head constantly telling you something—mostly negative. Take five minutes a day, and start writing about your inner chatter. What are you saying to yourself?

A great way to test your inner chatter is to pretend that the person speaking within your head is a person outside of your body. Spend five minutes every day with your new imaginary friend. Do you like what she has to say? Would you let your real friends speak to you like that? Most people find that when they engage in this exercise, they do not like their new imaginary friend at all. If the chatter is negative, the answer would be a resounding NO!

Another form of negative chatter is worry. When you worry or obsess about something in your life, you take up headspace that could be used for positive thoughts and actions. So many people get stuck in their lives because of endless worry and obsession cycles. Breaking the cycle and replacing those anxiety-producing thoughts with something different is the meaning of letting go. It's not easy to get rid of negativity, but knowing that we *can* get rid of it gives us hope for a brighter future. The reward of learning to *let go* is well worth the effort.

The good news is that only one thought can occupy your mind at any given time. If you are cognizant of your negative chatter, you can start changing it.

Start creating positive chatter; this may be as easy as writing down a few positive affirmations in a place where you can see them. Creating a vision board will be really helpful in replacing the negative thoughts with positive thoughts and goals. You can put anything you've ever dreamed of on your board, and I highly recommend just that.

Put it in a place that you can see every day. Physically seeing your vision board and visualizing what's on it will help you manifest it—help you actually achieve the goals you've set.

You can also create a vision board for each area of your life: one each for the person you want to be, the family you want to have, or the business you want to create. Some people have boards for becoming a better Christian or for obtaining the healthy body they desire.

Here's how you can create your vision board:

- Purchase a poster board (any size) of any color.
- Buy some magazines that you enjoy reading and that have something to do with the board you are creating.
- With a good attitude and an open mind, start cutting out pictures of what you enjoy, what brings a smile to your face, and what you wish to have.
- Do not censor yourself. Open your mind to the endless possibilities that life has to offer.

After analyzing your journal, preparing new goals, and creating your vision boards, you will notice a feeling of comfort. You now have what it takes to actually live the life God has intended for you. You are free to experience the love and joy you deserve. You are an amazing person, and your true happiness awaits!

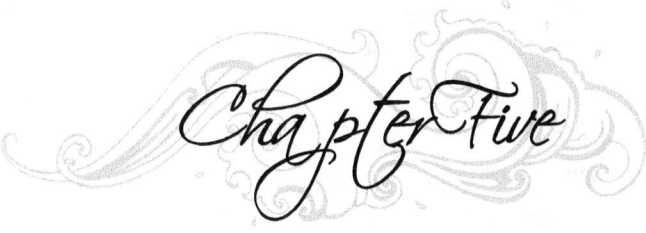

DRAW THE LINE

One of the most serious areas to look at as you analyze your journal is setting boundaries. Once you have your life plan in place, you will need to set boundaries to accomplish your goals. This is probably the hardest part of change, but is the most necessary.

Setting boundaries is about self-worth. So many of you, especially women, are brought up to be care-takers. A big part of making your life better is learning to love and respect yourself first. This means saying no at the right times and agreeing to terms that are right for you when necessary. This also means asking for help when you need it.

For many people, this will require a shift in consciousness. Part of respecting yourself is learning to treat others respectfully. Take stock of how you speak to the people around you. Do you nag? Do you yell at your spouse and children? Do you place more value in blaming instead of solving problems? Do you feel like people around you do not listen to you? These behaviors may all be the result of you working harder to change the people around you than changing your own behaviors to attract respect.

Why are setting boundaries so difficult? Mostly because of fear: fear that people won't like you if you stand your ground. Fear of changing the status quo in your life. Fear of retaliation. Fear that you might actually be successful. Yes, you read that correctly. Fear of what you might become should you actually make the changes you desire.

Boundary setting will require practice and you can expect resistance from some people in your life. When you start setting boundaries, you may notice that some people will become angry at you. Don't take it personally. Remember that as you are changing, the people around you will have to change as well if they want to remain a part of your life.

The toxic people will drop out of the picture and the people who respect you will remain. Don't feed into the anger of others about your change. Remain true to yourself and stick with your goals. The results will be amazing.

I know a woman who was divorced with two children. For years, she tried to keep family peace with an ex-husband who was verbally abusive and bad-mouthed her to anyone who would listen. One day, she decided enough was enough. Instead of "fighting fire with fire", as she used to call it, she decided to just be nice. Her ex started his barrage of insults (in front of their children), and she put up her hand and said, "I would appreciate it if you would speak to me respectfully, and, if you can't do that, do not speak to me at all. I do not deserve to be treated like this and will no longer tolerate it."

She said that everyone in the room stopped and stared at her like she was insane. After all, this had been going on for years. Her ex-husband pushed away the words and started in again, and she picked up her purse and left. This happened several times over the next couple of months.

She mentioned to me recently that she overheard a conversation between her daughter and ex-husband on the phone. Dad was berating his daughter about her play in a soccer event, and her daughter said, "Dad, I did the best I could, and I really would appreciate it if you would speak to me respectfully. If you can't do that, maybe you and I should take a break."

She was so proud of herself. Not only had she broken the exhausting and time-consuming cycle of behavior between her and her ex-husband, she'd also been able to teach her daughter a life-long lesson about setting her own boundaries.

Some boundary setting may make you feel guilty. This happens a lot when it comes to women and children. We live in a society where women are expected to be super-human. Don't feel guilty if you are not all things to all people.

Some mothers feel like they have to work all week and keep the perfect home. Let your teenage children clean their own rooms, and, if they won't, close the door! If you have a husband who throws his clothes on the floor and it drives you crazy to always be picking them up, stop picking them up. Walk over them, close your eyes when you walk by, and eventually he will do it himself.

Many of the overwhelming behaviors that we engage in are due to enabling the people around us. Analyze, without guilt, the tasks that you do for other people that they can do themselves. Just because they have become accustomed to you doing these tasks for them doesn't mean that you have to continue.

In order to set clear boundaries, you must name your limits. You cannot set good boundaries if you are unclear on where you stand. It is important to identify your emotional and spiritual limits. Consider what you will tolerate and accept. Also consider what makes you feel uncomfortable or stressed.

You must also be direct with the people around you. With most people, maintaining healthy boundaries requires you to have direct dialogue. People are not mind readers. Express your desires! People who understand the importance of setting boundaries respect themselves and should respect your boundaries too. Some people will require clear-cut communication, and you will need to be direct and concise about what you expect. You can expect some resistance and maybe even some hostility, but do not take their actions personally. People who are not taking your new boundary setting skills seriously may try to challenge them. The better prepared you are for this, the easier it will be for you to respond from a place of understanding, instead of defensiveness. Be sure to communicate your boundaries clearly to prevent disappointment. It is impossible for the people around you to know that you have new boundaries unless you actually communicate them. Be very precise and specific, so there is little to no miscommunication.

Communicate your new boundaries in a compassionate way. Let people know that you are doing things differently, but be respectful of their feelings as well. Walking into a room and announcing that you are "sick of everyone" and dumping this new way of doing things on them will not gain you the respect that you are looking for.

Fear, guilt, and self-doubt are all going to surface as you begin to set healthy boundaries. A pep talk will remind you that your boundaries are there to help you take back the life you deserve. Setting boundaries can be scary, but courage is important. Feel your fear, embrace your fear, and shove it out of the way, so you can move on with your life... your *happy* life!

Boundaries are all about acknowledging and honoring your feelings. If you find yourself slipping and not honoring the boundaries that you have set, ask yourself why. You gave yourself permission to have boundaries, now work to preserve them. Many times, we start letting boundaries slide because of pressure from others. Boundaries are not just signs of a healthy relationship, but also signs of self-respect. Remind yourself that your goal was self-respect. You cannot control what others do, but you can control how you treat yourself and how you respond to others.

Consider your past and your present needs as you set boundaries. Many of us were raised in families without role models who set boundaries. This is especially true in households where substance abuse took place. If you grew up in this type of environment, setting boundaries with your own family may be difficult. If you held the role of care-taker, you probably learned to focus more on the needs of others than your own. Ignoring your own needs might have become the norm for you. If this is the case, you may have to try setting one boundary at a time. Figure out which problem is the most pressing and work on that boundary first.

Taking care of yourself needs to become a priority. This means recognizing your feelings as important and honoring them. People may label you as "selfish" because you put your needs above theirs, but putting yourself first will create a sense of peace and well-being that is positive for everyone around you. Don't let other people guilt-trip you.

It is more important now than ever to seek support from others. Having a good support system as you start making these positive changes will help you stay focused on doing the best thing for you. If you are not comfortable sharing your emotions with any of your current friends, it would be helpful to talk to a counselor or someone from your church. You need your own cheering section to help you understand what a wonderful job you are doing, even when change doesn't feel so good.

It is not enough to just set boundaries. You have to stand up for yourself and enforce them. Be assertive with your needs. You will be challenged, so expect that and be strong. Stand up for your rights in a respectful way. If someone chooses to argue with you about your newfound self- respect, walk away without a fight. Arguing and being defensive about it takes your power away. Demand respect from others in a positive way, and always be respectful toward others. Follow the golden rule, "Do unto others as you'd have done unto you".

Setting and enforcing boundaries takes practice. Do not try to set ten new boundaries at once, or your life will be chaos. Start small, and choose one or two important areas to practice with first. Once you master those, move on to one or two more. The changes will be so dramatic that you will gain more confidence as you gain more skill.

It's time to take a stand for what you deserve. It's time to fight for what you want. It's time for a big change!

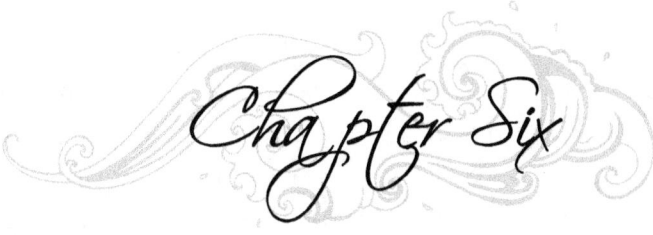

SELF-ACCEPTANCE

*D*ealing with your inner child and getting mentally healthy is the next step. Once you have your plan to move forward set in stone, you may find that some of the biggest obstacles exist within you.

In order to heal your inner child, you must first listen to it without being critical, overly demanding, or harsh. Many people reply to their negative self-talk in a tough way, especially when they feel afraid, anxious, or worthless.

The first step to healing your old wounds is to admit they're there. The next time you get a strange, uncomfortable, unwanted feeling, take the time to feel it and examine it. Write this awkward feeling down in your journal. Ask your inner child to explain the feeling to you. It takes a lot of courage to make this change, but once you learn how to talk to and nurture your inner child, you will find out many new things about yourself.

Many adults go day after day pretending that their inner child does not exist, or that everything is all right. They fool themselves into thinking they are too busy to stop and face that inner child. The healing process cannot take place if you ignore this aspect of yourself. As time goes on, old childhood patterns will continue to repeat themselves until they become so large that they can't be ignored.

An extreme example of this is the girl with "daddy issues." Typically, this will be a woman who is looking for love, because she didn't get enough from an emotionally distant father. Unfortunately, she looks for love and attracts the kind of man that she is familiar with, the emotionally distant man, over and over. Healing that wound will involve nurturing that little girl within her who didn't get enough love, and teaching her that she is worthy love from a man who is emotionally available.

A friend of mine had been divorced for nine years and was constantly complaining that he wanted a relationship. After listening to him complain for several years, I started to ask him some questions about his dating habits. His marriage ended because his wife cheated on him. I had always assumed that he didn't get involved in relationships, because he was afraid he would get hurt again. He said that women always left him.

The more I talked to him about this, the clearer it became that he was afraid of losing his independence.

He worked fifty-five hours a week and spent most weekends running ultras or cycling in races. Most of those weekends, he was out of town.

So I asked, "When do you date?"

He responded that he dated a couple times a month. He'd often take a woman out to dinner and go back to her house for sex afterwards.

His answer surprised me.

I asked if he spent the night or just left after sex.

He said he liked to wake up in his own bed, so he could get to work in the morning.

I was trying to be compassionate but laughed at him. I actually said, "These women let you get away with this?"

He said that most of the time he'd date someone for a couple months, and then she'd start to complain that he didn't spend enough time with her.

He disliked the complaining, so they'd drift apart.

From a distance, it's easy to see exactly why this man couldn't find the relationship he wanted so desperately. He didn't make time for a relationship.

After nine years, it had never occurred to him that the problem was not the women he chose. When I talked to him about what he wanted in a woman, he indicated that "convenience" was his top priority. He wanted someone he could call for dinner with little notice. He didn't realize that his definition of convenience was interchangeable with beck-and-call.

It never occurred to him that any worthwhile woman wouldn't be available at a moment's notice. As a result, he attracted needy women who would accept scraps of attention from him. No one was fulfilled. He was stuck in a vicious cycle that he'd created but blamed on others.

Relationships are not the only areas that your inner child may need to heal. People have habits and patterns that can extend into many other areas. Research is showing that many addictions are related to dysfunction in family structures. If you have a substance abuse problem, you will need to address this pattern before your life will get better. Most addicts start using to numb the pain that their inner child is experiencing.

Overcoming addiction is only the first step. Addictions are the result of many years of stuffing and numbing pain. Taking the substance away may cause many of those old feelings to surface, and without the substance to numb the pain, this can be a painful process.

The addictions that people recognize best are alcohol and drug related, but addictions like sex, Internet, and social media, are not as easy to spot. What about the obsession to be physically fit? An obsession with fitness can be used to avoid interacting with others on a more personal, intimate level.

If you don't recognize any of these addictions in your own life, be cognizant of their existence in the lives of those around you. These are red flags if you are dating or forming a friendship. Addiction translates into "emotionally unavailable" and you deserve a mate or friend who is emotionally available to you. The other end of that spectrum is "fixing." You need to know that a person with the addiction is the only person who can fix or change his own life. Don't put yourself in a position where you make a person like this a "project."

Research is finding that dysfunctional relationships are generational. It may be productive for you to analyze the family relationships in the home you grew up in. While doing this, remember to be forgiving toward the people who may not have treated you in a nurturing way. Remember that you can't change the past, and blaming your mother or father for your problems is not un-productive, but will do nothing to help you move forward.

Most parents do the best job they can under the circumstances. Analyzing your family relationships is about finding a way to heal and forgive. Healing yourself is the first step to breaking new ground with your own family and breaking the cycle of dysfunction.

Sometimes, healing your inner child can be done on your own with hard work. All your inner child is looking for is safety where previously there has been none. Provide the same nurturing environment that you would provide for your own children.

John Bradshaw, a leading expert on inner child work, describes the healing process as one of grief. In his book, *Home Coming: Reclaiming and Championing Your Inner Child,* he describes healing as a six-step process.

1. Trust

Your wounded child must come out of hiding. In order for him to do that, he must be able to trust that you will be there for him. Your inner child needs a supportive, non-shaming protector to validate his abandonment, neglect, enmeshment, or abuse. Those are the essential elements in original pain work.

2. Validation

You must take responsibility for what has happened in your past. This does not mean you are at fault, but you just need to recognize how you feel because of a past event and validate your feelings. Get in the habit of telling yourself, "I have the right to feel how I feel". This will help you work through your feelings much more easily, because you won't be so deeply embedded in the negativity about yourself.

3. Shock and Anger

If all of this is shocking and makes you angry, you have just entered the first stage of grief. It's okay to be angry, even if your wounds were inflicted unintentionally. In fact, you have to be angry if you want to heal your wounded inner child. Acknowledge to yourself that you are angry and have the power to choose to no longer tolerate the dysfunction and abuse in your own family system.

4. Sadness

After anger comes hurt and sadness. If you were victimized, you must grieve that betrayal. You must grieve for your unfulfilled developmental needs.

5. Remorse

When we grieve for someone who has passed away, remorse usually surfaces. We wish that we'd spent more time with the person who died. When we grieve for our inner child, it is the same, but his pain is about what happened to him, and we must remember we couldn't have done anything differently.

6. Loneliness

Toxic shame and loneliness represent the deepest of our feelings that are derived from grief. We are ashamed that we feel abandoned. We feel bad about ourselves, and that shame leads to loneliness. Since our inner child feels flawed, he has to cover up his true self with his false self. This false self is what he projects to others to hide the shame his true self feels. His true self becomes separated and remains alone and isolated.

Staying with this last layer of pain is the hardest part of the process. It is hard to stay with that level of shame and loneliness; but, as we embrace these feelings, we come out the other side and encounter that part of the self that has been hiding. The true healing lies in finding and nurturing that true self.

Many people cannot do all of this healing on their own. If you are in the throes of addiction, you may need rehab. If you are overwhelmed by the feelings that come to the surface when healing your inner child, you may need to engage the services of a licensed therapist, a pastor, or someone else who is experienced in guiding people through this process in a safe manner.

Regardless of how tough this process may be, it is absolutely necessary in order to detox your soul. Not only is it necessary, it is gratifying and satisfying! It feels amazing to confront your past in a healthy way. When you find the strength to face your fears and set healthy boundaries you finally have a clear vision to see your happy future. Your mind, body, and soul will appreciate this detox more than you know. Soon enough you will experience the life God intended for you!

Chapter Seven

BRAND NEW YOU

First of all, celebrate the fact that you have made this commitment to get your soul into shape. No more excuses! Your inner child has agreed that it's time, and you deserve to get your mind, body, and soul healthy. Something has finally clicked, and you are ready to create healthy habits that will last the rest of your life. Next, you will need to actually take some time to visualize what you want to physically look and feel like.

Sit in a quiet, comfortable place. Think of your fitness goal. Now, close your eyes, and imagine you got your "sexy" back! What do you look like? Imagine a fit and younger you. Imagine how much energy you have, how good you feel, and how much fun you are having!! The best way to stay focused on the person you want to be is to find an old picture of yourself when you felt you were at your best, or maybe even a picture of someone that inspires you. Put this picture on your refrigerator, so you are reminded of your goal every time you go to get something to eat or drink. Trust me! It will help you stay focused on your detox!

Here are a few general ideas to get you started:

Practicing healthy eating habits will go a long way toward helping you slim down, feel better, and live a longer, healthier life. This doesn't mean you must change everything or feel deprived. Even small changes will help you. Start by eating more vegetables and drinking more water. Getting your pH levels balanced are very important in detoxing your body. There is plenty of research showing the link between acidic pH and cancer. Cancer thrives in an acidic environment, and doesn't survive in a normal, more alkaline environment. Cancer cells make your body even more acidic as they produce lactic acid. Taking action to make your body more alkaline is vital in the battle against cancer. Unfortunately, the majority of the foods and drinks we consume are acidic, such as meat, grains, and sugar, with colas and other soft drinks being highly acidic. So unless you have been eating a very healthy diet, full of fresh fruit and vegetables, your body is way too acidic. Creating a very good environment in your body so that cancer cells cannot grow should be a major goal for you.

Make sure you drink more water. Filtered water helps remove toxins and will provide you with more energy for your activities. Since our bodies are about 60% water, try your best to consume at least 60% of your body weight in ounces of water every day. Keeping your body hydrated will help you maintain a healthy balance of your body fluids, which aid in digestion, absorption, circulation, creation of saliva, transportation of nutrients, and maintenance of body temperature.

Keeping your body hydrated allows it to function more efficiently. Even mild dehydration will slow down your metabolism as much as 30%. If you are dieting, one glass of water will shut down midnight hunger pangs.

If you exercise heavily or exercise in the heat, drink more water than normal. Also, drink a bottle of water *before* you work out. Many times, we think we need a bottle *while* we are working out but forget that our muscles should be hydrated *before* our workout. The water we drink during a workout is just for maintenance. Our muscles need water to stay energized.

Lack of water is also the number one trigger for daytime fatigue. It has been proven that 8-10 glasses of water per day can significantly ease back and joint pain, as well as decreasing the occurrence of many forms of cancer.

Eliminate a lot of sugar from your diet. Eating excess sugars can lead to diabetes and other diseases. Cancer feeds off sugar! It can also lead to sugar addiction. How many times have you reached for a candy bar when you are low on energy? Eating sugar may give you a short-term energy burst, but it can also make you crave more sugar. Not only will sugar make you fat, it can also set you up for sickness.

Try the sweetness of stevia, a natural herb found in your local health food store. Stevia will keep your blood sugar stable while aiding in fat loss. If your energy is low and you are craving sugar, reach for a handful of nuts instead. Nuts are high in protein and will reduce your cravings.

Eating small meals will also help you lose weight. Try to eat every 3-4 hours. Eating smaller meals throughout the day helps your metabolism to perform at its highest potential. This allows for quicker fat loss, keeps your mind sharp, and provides consistent energy throughout the day.

Eating frequently also helps eliminate cravings. If you work and cannot eat frequently, pack high protein snacks to eat on your breaks. Learn to eat until you are satisfied—and not until you've finished your entire meal. A good trick when eating out is to pack half of your plate to go as soon as you get it!

Eat lots of protein. Proteins are the building blocks of muscles, and they are made up of amino acids. Have protein at every meal.

Try a high-quality protein shake if you don't feel you are getting enough protein in your meals, or for a quick meal replacement. When buying a protein shake, be sure to look at the label and choose one that is low in sugar.

Good nutrition consists of a daily supply of amino acids in your diet, so that your body has the materials it needs to repair your muscles, organs, and other tissues. Eight amino acids are called the "essential amino acids" because they come from your daily diet. They are lysine, methionine, leucine, tryptophan, valine, phenylalanine, threonine, and isoleucine.

There are non-essential amino acids as well, which can be synthesized by the body and are different from those obtained by food. The term "non-essential" does not mean "less important." The human body is simply capable of creating non-essential amino acids on its own; therefore, it's unnecessary to obtain them from food.

Amino acids make up a lot of the human body and are vital to every part of human function. Meat, eggs, and dairy are the most common sources of these important building blocks. After strenuous exercise, your need for protein and amino acids rise. Protein drinks with amino acids are good to drink after a workout, because they increase the levels of amino acids in your blood and provide aminos that your body needs to build stronger muscles.

Your nervous system depends on amino acids to operate properly. If you lack the amino acid tryptophan, you may have lowered levels of serotonin, which may lead to depression and insomnia. New research shows that single aminos, or combinations of amino acids taken in capsule form, may help heal certain conditions. Glutamine has been proven to help curb alcohol or sugar cravings.

Eat raw foods every day. Raw foods are uncooked and unprocessed foods that give us energy. Choose organic for their incredible taste and to avoid unwanted pesticides and herbicides, which contain more toxins that our body needs to flush. Again, this is another reason to drink lots of water.

Eat right for your blood type. Your nutritional requirements are unique. Talk to your doctor or a nutritional counselor who can help you create healthier habits and tasty alternatives to fit your lifestyle.

The book, *Eat Right for Your Type*, by Peter J. D'Adamo, ND will help you establish a healthy diet just right for you.

Do not skip meals. If you skip meals, you may discover that you overeat at your next meal. This also causes your metabolism to slow down. If you are not a morning person, it may be difficult to get moving in the morning and have enough time to eat. Try buying protein bars or shakes, which are a good form of sustenance on the go, and snack on them on your way to work or the gym.

Look at the time of day at which you eat your meals. A common mistake is to eat dinner and then go to bed shortly afterward. Make sure you eat dinner early enough to burn off some of the calories. A good way to lose weight would be to limit carb intake in the afternoon and evening.

Exercise is also an important component of a healthy lifestyle. See your healthcare provider before beginning any form of cardiovascular exercise. People who are not in shape have a higher risk of getting hurt while doing high-intensity workouts.

If you currently do not exercise at all, start your regimen slowly. Week one should involve some sort of walk every day, even if it's only for 20 minutes. Daily exercise is very important. Not only is it helpful when trying to lose weight, but it also keeps your mind and soul healthy.

After week one, aim for three to five days of cardio training for 20 to 60 minutes, as recommended by the American College of Sports Medicine. Eventually, you should be working out for an hour every day, even if it's just walking for that hour. It's amazing how good you feel when you look good, too!

Exercising too soon after a full meal can compromise oxygen and nutrient delivery to your working muscles (where you need it). Also, remember to drink water before, during, and after working out. Take extra water with you if you exercise outdoors.

Always start with a warm-up and end with a cool-down for five to 10 minutes at a low intensity. Stretch before, during, and after exercise. This will help improve your post-workout recovery, keeping you pain-free with higher amounts of energy.

Maintain your heart rate at the Healthy Heart Zone. Talk to your doctor about your individual numbers.

Aerobic exercise is great, but you also need a weight training program. Recruit a good personal trainer who can save you time by tailoring a fitness program to get you fast results safely. Most gyms offer a personal trainer to discuss your needs and goals when you join. Take advantage of this service.

Start with light weights. The tendency to use too much weight typically results in poor form and reduces your ability to get results while increasing the risk of injury.

Be sure to use slow, controlled movements. Lifting weights fast and out of control will not only cause injury, but will thwart your efforts to get results. Do not judge yourself because you are only using a 10 lb. weight. It is WAY more important to better your form, than sustain an injury. If you find yourself bored or unchallenged by weight training, change your fitness routine. By changing your routine every six weeks, you continue to challenge the body to keep progressing. No need to revamp the entire workout—just changing a few exercises will help prevent you from reaching those dreadful plateaus.

Avoid over-training. Never train the same muscle group two days in a row, except your abdominal muscles. You can do as many sit-ups as you can tolerate daily! For instance, I make sure to work different muscle groups every day. Mondays, I work biceps and back. Tuesdays, I work triceps and chest. Wednesday is leg day and cardio only. Thursday is usually shoulders only this day. Friday is just cardio, and Saturday I combine some exercises from each core muscle group. I work my abs every day, and I try to run at least a mile every day, except Sunday. Sunday is REST DAY. Signs of overtraining are feeling burnt out, weak, and/or sore. If you do over-train and feel sore, drink more water than usual.

Core strengthening is also key for maintaining a healthy body. While experts differ on which muscles make up the core muscles, most target the region of your body that includes the length of the trunk and torso. These muscles are responsible for stabilizing the spine and pelvis.

The benefits of good core strength range from reducing back pain to improving postural imbalances. The abdominal muscles are responsible for protecting the back muscles; weak core muscles are the primary source of lower back pain. Because the muscles of the trunk and torso stabilize the spine, training these muscles can also lessen sports-related injuries.

If you want a good, all-around workout that involves your core, start with a Pilates class. Pilates is a body conditioning system that will help build flexibility and muscle strength in the legs, abdominals, hips, and back, putting emphasis on pelvic and spinal alignment, breathing, and developing a strong core. Pilates improves muscle tone, posture, and teaches moves with grace and ease.

Yoga is also a good all-body workout. It brings the mind, body, and spirit together by stretching the body into different poses while keeping breathing controlled. While many view Yoga as an exercise, this practice can also be used to bring a feeling of connectedness with God.

Studies have shown that Yoga relieves stress, reduces cortisol levels, improves sleep, lowers blood pressure, and can improve many medical symptoms. Other benefits include increased strength and flexibility, reduced anxiety and muscle tension, and spiritual growth.

If you have a limited amount of time in your life for exercise, spiritual commitment, and stress relief, Yoga may be a one-stop solution. Most cities have a yoga studio or spa and many gyms offer yoga classes, so it should be easy to locate a place near you.

Whether you start with walking, Pilates, or Yoga, aim for something you enjoy. Even just 20 minutes a day exercising with a friend will make a huge difference in your quest to detox your soul. Your life will be better, and most likely longer, when you eat healthy and exercise. It's relatively simple, but takes time and dedication. We all have to start somewhere. Why not today?

Chapter Eight

SHAPING YOUR SPIRIT

$\mathcal{N}$ow that your body is on its way to becoming healthy, it's time to get your spirit in shape, too! Becoming spiritually healthy is simply a matter of learning certain spiritual exercises. Just like getting physically fit requires exercise, we must become self-disciplined in our spiritual lives. Meditation is a good way to get closer to God and develop a strong sense of spirituality. Meditation is the art of focusing 100% of your attention to one area. Meditation doesn't have to be some long, drawn-out ordeal. It can be a simple as taking 10 minutes to yourself and just laying on your bed, closing your eyes, and taking deep breaths. Just focus on your breathing, and RELAX! This may seem easy, but it can be very difficult for some people. You may feel uncomfortable, and negative thoughts may surface. Just continue to focus on your breathing, and it will eventually become second nature to you. Meditation is a wonderful practice that will help you detox your soul!

Taking the time to develop good spiritual habits helps shape good character traits. In order to develop spiritual fitness, our daily habits must include time spent with God, prayer, Bible reading, and obedience to what He reveals.

This isn't something that will happen quickly. Our society is one that feeds off instant gratification.

I used to have a license plate frame that said "I want it all and I want it now." That was the attitude I had. It took me a *long* time to figure out how much God's word fulfilled me, and that I didn't need *it all*, and I certainly didn't need it *now*.

This self-discovery has been a very gradual process for me. For some of you who grew up with God's arms around you and never strayed from that place, this is easy for you. For those who have taken unrighteous paths, this may be a tougher task. And for those of you who have never felt God's unconditional love, this may be the toughest, yet most rewarding, thing you have ever done in your life.

Nobody should expect to throw his or her soul in the microwave and nuke it with God's love. Once you commit your life to Jesus, you're *immediately* guaranteed everlasting life in Heaven, but growing spiritually is a gradual process—a lifetime endeavor. It takes patience. God continually changes us. He will help us achieve those results we so desire, but we must show Him that we are truly ready.

We can't pray for more money, but then be horrible money managers. It doesn't work that way. If you learn to manage your money in a way that would make God happy, He will bless you beyond belief! Same with anything else! If you continually pray to get rid of the negative people in your life, but still choose to hang out with them, that's not God's fault. He gives us all free will, and the paths we choose to head down are 100% our responsibility.

The point of my earlier story about an "instant gratification society" is that people who have strong spiritual beliefs do not need to have everything now. They trust in God to bring them the things that they want with the timing that is necessary.

Trusting in this is a huge test for all of us because it means having the virtue of patience and believing that everything in our lives happens for a reason. It is giving up control in a way that honors God.

When we take a good look at the instant gratification society, what do we see? We find people who will do anything in the name of greed. They will walk over the rights of others, steal to get ahead, and, in some cases, even physically hurt others to get what they want.

That sort of behavior cannot enrich the soul. In fact it is destroying it.

What also stands out is the quality of communication in an instant gratification society. Daily, I see couples who meet on the Internet and jump into relationships. These relationships fizzle as fast as they burned, because they have not been nurtured.

Part of spiritual fitness is the ability to walk away from instant gratification. If you date, know your value and the value of getting to know someone before making a commitment to them. As Christians, sex should not even be an issue until marriage, yet so many women feel that they have to take part in instant intimacy or a man will leave them. Trust that God has someone better in mind who will respect your wishes—and let the other people go.

Setting boundaries involves making a commitment to ideals that help us make our spiritual life richer. One of those commitments should be to eliminating junk moods. Junk moods are the people, places, and things in your life that drain your energy or entrap you in negative moods. Getting rid of these extraneous items that create chaos in your life will help you achieve balance, peace, and connectedness to you soul.

To eliminate junk moods, have a plan of action to bring you back to a place of peace. For example, doing something nice for someone else when you start to feel negative will make someone else feel good and lift your spirits as well. This can be something as simple as holding the door for someone or smiling at a stranger. Expressing gratitude or complimenting someone else can also uplift both you and others. Random acts of kindness bring peace and joy to us all. The world needs more of this, and you can be the start.

As you explore your spiritual personality, take a few minutes to write down in your journal the things that bring you peace, connection, and joy. This might also be a good time to start a new spiritual practice. Could you take a half hour out of every day to journal, meditate, or pray? Remember that the best spiritual practice is whatever brings you closer to Jesus. Don't be afraid to try new spiritual practices. If something brings you peace, incorporate it into your routine. If it doesn't work, consider it a learning experience.

New spiritual practices present the opportunity to explore the mind and body connection. Make a list of the areas of your body where you have intermittent or chronic pain. Many times, these areas are where you hold your stress.

Here are a few tips and ideas:

1. Figure out what your main problem is and write it down. Is your boss treating you unfairly? Is a co-worker harassing you? Is your teacher too hard on you? Is your classmate bullying you? Is your spouse cheating on you? Are your kids driving you crazy?

2. Think about what you have done so far. What actions have you taken to try and solve this problem on your own? No one is interested in helping someone who will not help themselves, so it is a good idea to define what steps you have taken on your own to tackle the problem. Sometimes, you may figure out another possible solution you hadn't thought of yet.

3. Reflect on what you can actually control. Remember, you cannot control other people's feelings or actions, so it wouldn't be worth your while to spend your energy trying. If you are being bullied,

you cannot control the bully's behavior, but you *can* control how you respond to their words and actions. Knowing the difference between what you can and cannot control will help you see ways in which other people may be able to help you with your problems.

4. Define your expectations. What specifically can someone else do to help you with your issue? If the problem is bullying, maybe you could ask a teacher to move your desk away from the person who is picking on you. This way, you are a part of the solution. *You are the solution.* Be realistic in your expectations—you cannot ask someone else to do something that is beyond their scope of control any more than you can expect yourself to do those things.

5. Ask and have courage. Realize that you *deserve* help. Know that asking isn't a sign of any weakness, as you may have told yourself in the past. Remain positive but assertive when asking for help to let the other person know you are serious and being realistic in your expectations. It may help to share what you have already done, as well as your understanding of the things beyond your control. If someone rejects your request for help, realize they are rejecting a request, not rejecting you. This is when you need to remember you are an amazing person with lots of great qualities. This is when you remember that not everyone is capable of helping you. This is when you just simply say "thank you" and move on to someone else who can. Don't give up! Keep asking until you find help!

Approaching every situation with a positive attitude will help you, no matter what! Praying about the issue will help give you clarity and give you the strength and patience to resolve it. With God's help you will succeed!

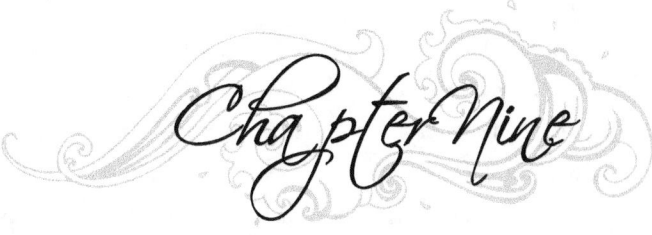

HELP WANTED:

Letting your guard down and being vulnerable is one of the hardest things to do. In this world of advanced technology, everyone is connected, and the world moves at a rapid pace. Many people feel that they have to be the best at everything and do it all. Look at how crazy our world has become for our children who play sports. Not only is the child having to practice several days a week, they are on traveling teams and play in tournaments. The parents are pushing their kids to be the best, and sometimes fighting with other parents in the stands. Some people have lost all sense of what's best for their children. They are caught up in "being the best" and having the "best" kids in the world. These people spend more time focusing on being the best rather than doing what really is best. It's really okay to not be the best. It's really okay if your kid isn't the star player on his team. It's okay to just *slow down*. God has a wonderful plan for each and every one of us, and, if we continue to make choices that do not please Him, then we will continue to suffer. Focus on God and your family and all things will fall into place as they should. It's tough enough to admit when you need help, but asking for help is even harder. Learning to be your own advocate is one of the most important things you can do for yourself. Every one of us is unique and worthy of love, respect, and assistance from others. But for some of us, it's extremely difficult, and sometimes even painful, to admit what we need.

Developing the skills to ask for help takes time, patience, and lots of practice. It can be very uncomfortable, but, if you have the courage to ask, you will find that a great burden can be lifted.

People may not want to appear weak, needy, or incompetent, but the danger of not asking for help is that a small problem can grow into a crisis when it is ignored.

Generally men have a harder time letting their guard down than women, because many men have the "caveman syndrome". A lot of men need to feel they are the sole provider for their family, which is truly what God intended anyhow. Unfortunately, we live in a society that demands that everyone work hard.

The changed social norms include women working more, and being home less often, although some men still expect their partners to solely care for the kids and the house. The Bible says women are to be the man's "helper", but it takes working together to create the rules of the family household and expectations for the relationship.

Many churches offer marriage classes, which you may find useful, whether you are planning a wedding or have been married for years. Once you both know the ground rules for how a loving, Christian marriage should work, it's much easier to make a game plan for a great future together.

One major issue remains that many people still think they can solve all problems on their own. If we all clearly established our roles and responsibilities early on, and worked from the same expectations, there wouldn't be so much animosity later. Communication is key!

Some people fear losing control, which may result in their being hurt—emotionally or physically. Many people don't want to feel indebted to another person. Asking for help can shift the power in a relationship, which can be a scary prospect if you think the other person may take advantage of you. This is where learning to be your own advocate can be your best course of action.

Being your own advocate means putting yourself first. This is not to be confused with being selfish, but instead should be recognized as making a commitment to be authentic with each decision.

Always try to ask for help in a reciprocal sense: "If you can take my child to school today, I will pick yours up next week." Be sure to hold up your end of the bargain. Nothing makes people more resentful than feeling they have been taken advantage of.

Be sure that you always engage someone who will reciprocate. You do not want to continually have someone come to your aid who wants nothing in return. The imbalance of that relationship can make everyone uncomfortable. Having integrity is one of the most important aspects of life. Do what you say and say what you mean.

If you're not used to asking for help, here are some clear rules:

1. Be straightforward and assertive in a nice respectful way.
2. When you turn a project or task over to someone, do not micromanage. Let it go and have faith.
3. If possible, make your request in person. Texts and emails seem to be harsh to others and can often be misinterpreted.
4. Be sure to thank the person immediately after you strike the deal.

Sometimes we are overwhelmed and need the help of an organization or support group to pull us from our denial and confront some real truths. We need to recognize that our need for help only allows our soul to be replenished. It feels great when we achieve a goal, especially when others have assisted in the process. Celebrate those victories, whether big or small, and always show your appreciation to those who have helped you along the way. Who knows? Maybe that person may need help to detox their soul someday too!

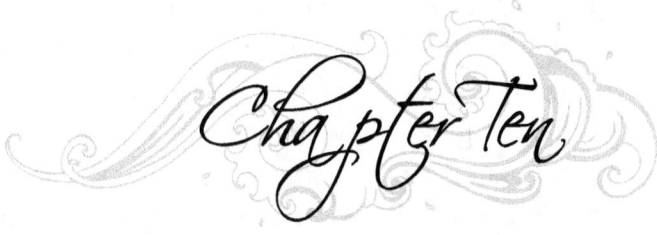

THE ENABLER

$\mathcal{I}$s your life more complicated because you are enabling someone who has a dependency problem? Is your life on unsteady ground? You may need to address some deep problems within yourself that are holding you back. Before you can connect with yourself and your soul on any intimate level, you will need to evaluate these questions.

Is your life hectic and chaotic because you have a spouse who is an alcoholic or does drugs? In many families, this is a secret that no one talks about or acknowledges. It may feel shameful to admit that you or someone close to you may have an out-of-control problem. The addiction may not be something that the entire family sees on a daily basis.

Some people have addictions that are not as easy to spot, such as pornography or gambling. Are you still expecting this person to change without help? Is he or she refusing help?

Should you talk to someone at church about this issue? Should you have an intervention? Should you take the kids and stay at your parents for a while? These are all questions that you need to pray about. If you or your children are in danger, the answer is pretty clear. You need to get away and separate your children and yourself from the addict for the good of the family. It is important that you get help from your church or city authorities.

Separation may include cutting off funding to a gambler and delivering ultimatums that protect your own boundaries. If you are involved with an addict who is violent under the influence, you may have to consider pressing criminal charges. If there is no present danger, but you feel there may be in future, you need to set clear boundaries. If the boundaries are not respected, it's time do to something different.

If you are the person who needs help, but you are too ashamed to ask, there are many organizations out there that can help you. If you have a dependency problem, Alcoholics Anonymous, Narcotics Anonymous, or even your church may be the best place to start. Your church may have a Celebrate Recovery program, which is a wonderful way to get started on the road to recovery.

If a loved one has a problem but won't seek help, Alcoholics Anonymous may be a place for you to get support. This program will allow you to seek help from people who are also going through the same thing.

Please know that none of this will be easy. Most addicts suppress their feelings because they are too painful to confront. Quitting their drug of choice will make them feel those things they've suppressed for a very long time.

Change doesn't happen overnight. You will find that as you change the dynamic of your life, others around you will react. Many times, the reaction will not be favorable. Remember, as difficult as it is for you to change, it is just as difficult for those around you.

As you start asking friends and family for help, they may resent your "rocking the boat" for a time, but know that the end result of the new you will be worth it.

Have the courage to ask for help and the faith to know that the help will get you one step closer to becoming the person you really want to be.

Praise and thanks daily to our Lord will help you find the peace and patience you will need during this tough time.

Remember, a road without obstacles is probably one that doesn't lead to where you want to be.

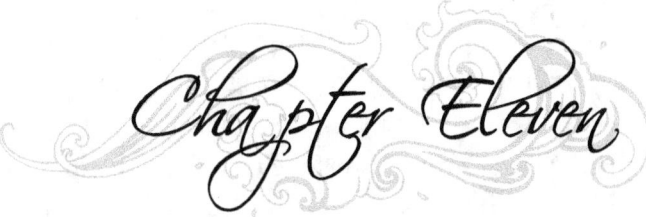

CHANGE YOUR THOUGHTS; CHANGE YOUR LIFE

$\mathcal{W}$e all have the opportunity to interpret our reality. We interact with, react to, avoid, and enjoy God's creation we call life. This means that we have the ability to look at a situation and see both sides, which gives us options—the option to choose the positive or the negative. Positive thoughts create more positive circumstances. Conversely, negative thoughts contribute to negative feelings, such as unhappiness or disillusionment.

Changing your thoughts from negative to positive will change the course of your life. If you choose to stay stuck in the negative thought process, your life will change too, but for the worse.

Many people do not know how to make the transformation immediately from thinking negatively to thinking positively. One tip is to stay away from all-or-nothing thinking.

Do you know someone who thinks in all-or-nothing terms? The world is black and white; there are no shades gray. This kind of thinking limits our possibilities. People who lead emotionally balanced lives are flexible. Black-and-white thinking leaves little room for interpretation and can be a rigid place to live.

How do you know you are rigid? Look at the way you speak to others. Words are a powerful clue to how flexible you are. Words like *impossible, terrible, never,* and *always* are good examples of words that communicate an attitude of powerlessness.

Positive people take responsibility for their lives, and powerlessness is not a part of their vocabulary.

Do you know someone who is so stubborn that they self-sabotage? The need to be *right* cultivates negative thoughts and destroys relationships.

How do you eliminate this from your life? Make a decision to be happy instead of right.

If you argue with your spouse, kiss and make up before you go to bed. Agree to disagree and forgive easily. This brings us back to the power of words. If you disagree with someone in your life, use your words carefully. Don't say something that you will regret later. Keep in mind that once something comes out of your mouth, it can never be fully taken back. And if you do hurt someone with your words, be sure to apologize sincerely as soon as possible.

I like to use the analogy of a broken plate. You can glue it back together, but it will never be the same. Relationships are just like that.

Changing your mental filter is one of the keys to a positive life. Letting chronic, negative thinking creep into our consciousness is easy, but try to make a conscious effort to see the world as a glass half-full.

Jumping to conclusions is a common negative trap. When a situation presents itself that seems negative, be patient, take a deep breath and a step back and get all of the information before you react.

When you are ready to react, try reacting in the most positive way possible. You will be amazed at how *everyone* involved will feel better.

Life should not be about hurting others, but instead about being more understanding and forgiving. God calls us to love our enemies, yet this is one of the hardest things to do. Doing this is the best for *you*, because you no longer have to carry any of that hurt or resentment in your heart. You control your feelings!

This may come as a surprise, but everything is not all about you. Why am I telling you this? Because many people take their lives so seriously that they are very easily offended.

When you feel like you are taking a situation personally, take a step back and think about it for a moment before responding.

Sometimes someone's negative comment means that he or she is just having a bad day or is just plain insensitive. Have enough self-esteem to be able to let things slide. This does not mean that you should take abuse from someone chronically, just that sometimes their negativity is about them and not you.

Let's talk about drama. When we are involved in a negative situation, it is easy to magnify the problem and make it much larger than it needs to be. Drama feeds the negative problem and blows it out of proportion (perception). Seeing the problem for what it is (reality) will allow you to become grounded and treat it accordingly.

Ungrounded people magnify problems and give them more energy, which ends up draining them and the people around them. I have watched a mother yell at her ex-husband and his new wife after a parent teacher conference. Knowing the full story, I know this woman's rage stems from her jealousy of her ex-husband's new wife, but the drama she creates all the time isn't good for anyone. It's best to walk away or not even allow yourself to be put in these types of situations.

Feed your positive outlook by celebrating the good things that happen. We all have setbacks and obstacles. There are days when we will be sad and drained. By celebrating the good days, we will begin to notice more we can be grateful for and fewer obstacles.

Now that you are on a course-correction toward a positive life, what about those negative people around you?

For the purposes of this discussion, we will label them "toxic friends."

How do you identify toxic people in your life? The easy answer is that you no longer feel good around them. Here are some signs to ponder:

You no longer feel comfortable when you are with this person.

You feel anxious or afraid when you receive communication from this person.

You have a nagging feeling that this person is not behaving genuinely and wants something from you.

After spending time together, you feel drained, tired, or stressed out.

You feel put down or inferior in the presence of this person.

If you have someone in your life who leaves you with any of these feelings, it may be time to analyze the relationship further.

There are several types of toxic friends. If your friend fits into one of these categories, it may be time to let them go.

The Opportunist: This person is in your life to further his or her own agenda. They don't respect or care about you. They only like you because you have a nice car or a big house. Or, they might be using you to get close to your friends or family. This person becomes angry when you confront them.

The Narcissist: This person lives by the mantra, "It's all about me". They always talk about themselves. They don't seem to care about you, how you are feeling, or how your day went. They also brag a lot and have an opinion about everything.

The Gossiper: This friend thrives on scandal and drama. She says something negative about most everyone. Be careful with this one;

if she says these things about others, chances are she does the same thing behind your back.

The Cling-On: This person wants whatever you have. Most often, this person is jealous of what you have, because of his or her own insecurities. This person also doesn't like to share you. When they see you with others, they act jealous, because they want you all to themselves. The strange thing is, if they are married or have a significant other, they will never include you to hang out with them. But when that person is busy, they want you during that time and yet will gladly ditch you for their significant other.

The Victim: This person only contacts you when there is something wrong. When all is good, he or she disappears. If you listen carefully, you may notice no acknowledgment of any personal responsibility for the bad situation. They typically stay mad at you after an argument, because they only accept their point of view. This person is a powerless victim, and may need a good therapist. Remember you are not their therapist, so don't let them air their grievances at your expense. It is important to show you care, but not involve yourself too much so that if affects your own life.

The Fake: This person will smile at your face, but will have no problem putting you down in front of others. They may also do drugs or have other bad habits, but will deny it. They promise to call you or help you, but never do. They always keep you waiting and make excuse after excuse.

Now that you have identified your toxic friends, it is time to eliminate them from your circle. Dumping friends can be a difficult proposition. Many people feel guilty about this task. Don't let guilt take over. You need to remind yourself that you are worth it and you deserve people who bring out your best qualities.

Do you know someone who thinks "inside the box" all the time? That kind of person is set in their ways and seems to do everything the same exact way daily.

Do you become frustrated when dealing with this person? What makes you feel frustrated?

Taking a look at our own thoughts makes us realize that *our thoughts* frustrate us, not that person's actions. If we learn to control our thoughts, and start thinking more positively, *we* will experience the life we really want. It's time to gain control.

You may decide to change your thoughts, or you may even decide that this person's behavior is toxic and unhealthy to be around. And that's okay. We all need to stop feeling guilty for wanting to weed out negative influences on our life.

If you stop saying to yourself "I feel horrible for thinking about telling this person I can no longer be friends with them", and start saying "I feel amazing that I am choosing to give myself a better life by not being friends with this person with toxic behavior", then you will feel amazing!

How much better would you feel thinking the *positive* thought? Spend time praying for this person. Ask God to grant them the peace and love they deserve. You never know what that person is really going through, so soften your heart enough to pray for them. We all need to do a better job loving our enemies!

By learning to set boundaries, you have the ability to say no to toxic people. Start to say no—no to receiving distress texts, no to family members who are behaving rudely, no to everyone who is negative.

Recently, a couple of my high school friends came back into my life. At first, I was happy to reconnect.

But then I started to realize that one of them, in particular, was a problem. She was an alcoholic and relied on rides everywhere so that she would not drink and drive. She would call me and ask me to go someplace with her, and I would drive half an hour out of my way to pick her up.

We would arrive at our destination, and she would drink too much and complain about her marriage for hours.

As you can imagine, an evening with her was exhausting. I soon started to say no to going out with her.

Unexpectedly, a mutual friend stated saying things to me about not picking up my end of the "driving chores." I was appalled and politely let her know that I was not interested in enabling our friend's drinking problem.

Both people took offense to this and haven't invited me out since. I felt bad for a few days, and then I realized there was a reason I quit hanging around with them years ago. I then felt powerful in my own decision. I was comforted with the fact that I was helping myself, and hopefully them as well.

You can't help someone who doesn't want to change. Don't let them drag you down too. Do not push anyone to change. Say what you feel and the rest is up to them.

If saying no isn't enough, you will have to speak to them directly about the problem—politely and with compassion for their feelings.

Start by speaking honestly about your feelings. By using "I feel" statements, you cannot be wrong, because you feel how you feel, and that is important. You need to stand up for yourself, but the goal should be to remain cordial.

If, during your talk, the other person becomes defensive, abusive, or blaming, this may be a sign that the relationship is not salvageable. Walk away and know that you tried your best.

You may just have to tell the person directly that you do not wish to be friends anymore. While this seems cruel, sometimes your honesty is the best thing you can offer.

Sometimes when a person breaks off a relationship, he or she will say they want to remain friends—but rarely is this true. Some people do this to stay connected so they can string you along. If you have been on the receiving end of this statement after a break-up, the most loving thing you can do for yourself is to clearly and calmly articulate that you cannot be friends.

Your first priority is healing from your heartbreak. If you are meant to be friends, this may happen later on after you have healed and moved on with your life. Love yourself enough to be clear.

Is it okay to just disappear from a toxic person's life? Yes it is, but only as a last resort. Abandoning someone without a reason that has been articulated is unkind. If you repeatedly turn down invitations, they will get the message; however, you should always give the other person an opportunity to improve, and speaking with them honestly will provide them with the knowledge to choose.

Not only are some of our friends and family members toxic, but we sometimes are toxic to others. We are all guilty of pouring our hearts out to another person, which is okay as long as it doesn't cross the line.

Set clear boundaries with yourself. If you have a problem that seems overwhelming, unburden yourself in the presence of a professional who will listen and guide you through the healing process.

It's good to talk about normal problems with your friends, but if you constantly talk about your "horrible" marriage, or your "destructive" relationship, or your "mis-behaved" children, you will lose your friends.

Better to find the time to *solve* the issues you need to talk about. A good marriage or family therapist could be very helpful for tough circumstances. Pray about these issues, and try talking to a Pastor at Church.

Many people have the misconception that "if you are in therapy, you must be a psycho." This is the furthest thing from the truth. People are constantly going to the doctor when they don't feel well physically, so why not go see a therapist when your emotions need help? Trust me, it works!

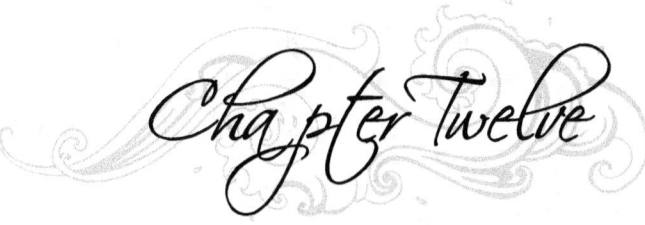

TRUE INTIMACY

*M*any of us dream of finding a soul mate, yet instant gratification seems to be at the center of today's dating patterns. Many adults use the term *sex* interchangeably with *intimacy*.

They are not one and the same.

Intimacy can be physical, emotional, intellectual, or spiritual. One of the main ingredients to being intimate is having a strong sense of self. Without this, you can't have a healthy, committed relationship.

A strong sense of self, starts with building a solid and strong boundary. Relationships require flexibility, compromise, and consideration. You and your partner should have a say in decisions that impact both of your lives; however, intimate partnerships also need space, not to keep your partner away, but to keep your identities intact while being together.

You should never feel like you have to discard essential parts of yourself to be in a relationship.

You might be asking how to remain true to yourself while being committed to your partnership. The answer is to take your time and get to know your potential partner.

Many people still struggle with the concept that we should be married before we have sex, but that is what God demands of us. It's no wonder that so many relationships end up failing when people use sex as a way to form a good relationship. The opposite is true: a good relationship will form good sex!

A relationship should have the following ingredients before engaging in sex:

- Respect
- Good communication
- Independent thoughts and activities as individuals
- Mutual support
- Commitment to the relationship
- MARRIAGE

Being in an intimate relationship is a wonderful opportunity for personal growth. It is a venue for working towards a long-term relationship, some merging of interests and activities, and even a merging of personalities. Every step in the growth process should be embraced for internal reasons, without external pressures. Most importantly, the changes should be gradual.

If you are looking at a potential partner, you need to spend enough time to spot problems that indicate that one or both of you has poor boundaries. If you are married and now spot major issues, it may be time for therapy. Ignoring the problems or fighting about them isn't healthy.

If you are with a partner who tells you that he has no idea what he or she wants, it is time to take a step back and give that person space while you continue your search for a partner. If your spouse is saying this, again, therapy will help!

Do not take this personally or think that you failed. Just keep that positive thinking and tell yourself you are "one step closer to THE ONE," or "I deserve love and respect in this marriage".

Another clue that you or your partner may not have a clear sense of self is when one of you engages in limiting behavior. For instance, a man who makes major decisions for you may be someone who is controlling.

Letting your partner deny you sufficient time alone or with your family and friends is cause for a new boundary or a break-up.

If you are married to someone like this, you need to establish clear, healthy boundaries, so you can enjoy the life you are meant to have. A jealous streak may be romantic in the movies, but in real life it is a sign of insecurity and usually causes more hurt.

If you find yourself altering your own hobbies, interests, and friends to match your partner's, reconsider the value of being yourself! Acting contrary to your own values or succumbing to pressure from your partner to change your appearance or engage in sexual activities that you are not comfortable with is never in your best self-interest.

Setting boundaries with your partner needs to be done on a regular basis. If your boundaries have been lacking, good communication is necessary to bring them back into focus for both of you.

If you have been enabling a behavior, you need to take responsibility and have a conversation about better boundaries.

If you are the one who has been engaging in unhealthy boundaries, you need to take responsibility for that as well, adjust, and strive to work on the issue.

A good sense of balance is necessary to endure a healthy relationship. Figure out what both of your needs are, compromise on a few things, and establish healthy boundaries together. You will soon realize how rewarding this can be!

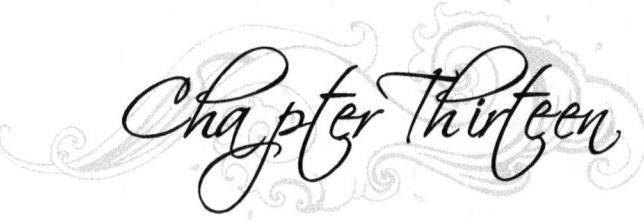

THERE'S AN APP FOR THAT

$\mathcal{T}$he purpose of this chapter is to bring your awareness to the positive points in your life. By now, you have worked on breaking habits that have held you back from having the life you've always wanted. Now that you have freed up the space that was filled with negativity, you have room to fill it with positive thinking and the manifestation of the desires you have always reached for.

It is not easy to shift your consciousness. The suggestions below are ways to focus your awareness towards one concept as a goal for the day.

As you become more disciplined, you will find that you are able to set goals that you can achieve. You will also find that you are replacing your old unhealthy habits with new healthy practices.

Here is a monthly calendar app for you to follow to help establish your new "detoxed soul".

Day 1 "A Fresh Start" - Wake up one hour earlier than normal. Spend some time meditating or reading the Bible, and then take a walk or get some exercise. Pack a *healthy* lunch and maybe a few healthy snacks. Eating healthily is important and can make you feel so much better about yourself. Take a walk in a new area of town. You never know what wonders lie in your city until you really take some time to explore and let your mind wander.

Day 2 "Me Time" - Shut down. Turn off your phone. At least once a day, preferably before bedtime, create a peaceful moment where you can be alone and take time to breathe deeply, meditate, pray, or just sit quietly. Clear your mind and bring closure to the events of the day while preparing for a restful night's sleep. Inhale slowly and visualize things to release from your mind's space. When you exhale, see those items coming out of your mind and spirit in that breath as you truly let go. Give thanks to God for all His glory!

Day 3 "Thanksgiving" - Instead of spending time engaging with potentially negative co-workers or friends, call a family member that you haven't talked to in a while and talk about the "good ol' days". On your way home from work, stop and buy some flowers. Put the flowers in the vase that you use for special occasions, and then make yourself a healthy dinner. Before you go to bed, kneel down beside your bed and give thanks to God for all the blessings in your life.

Day 4 "Let it Out" - We all must release some tears to help shed the layers that prevent us from growing in every aspect of life. Learn the value in the storms that test you. Don't be afraid to weep. A silent cry never hurt anyone—it simply cleanses your spirit and helps you move on. Crying can be an empowering experience, if you let it. It's ok to be sad, mad or hurt and it's ok to express these emotions. Don't hold it all in, or you will explode with anger someday! Give thanks to God that you are able to experience all the trials and tribulations in your life, and that you are stronger today because of them.

Day 5 "Throw It Down" - Have a problem in your life? Feeling frustrated about something? Write it down. Put all your worries on paper, and write about what's really on your mind. Whether you are angry with someone, or are simply experiencing an internal conflict, write it all down, and then shred the paper. Rip it up and throw it away just like the worries you wrote down. Make a chart to stay organized and keep track of how you can better yourself. It takes a lot of strength to realize what your internal conflicts are, because no one is perfect. Thank God for all that you have!

Day 6 "Beautiful Day" - Focus on your positives and believe in your beauty! Loving what you see is one of the most powerful lessons you can learn. Losing your fears and inhibitions requires loving yourself completely and stretching out of your comfort zone. God made you perfect just the way you are, so visualize yourself as a knockout. You are who you think you are. Remember, beauty is a state of mind, and, if you believe it, you will achieve it. Thank the Lord for giving you free will. Pray that you start using it more wisely.

Day 7 "Give Back" - Do something nice for someone today. Don't expect anything in return. The best way to increase your blessings is to do an unselfish act for someone else. Do something as simple as giving a homeless person a burger from McDonald's, or a one dollar bill. Offer to watch your neighbor's kids for the night, so they can enjoy a nice evening together. Call your local city planning department and ask if they need help. Helping the community feels good. Volunteer at your local food drive or community shelter. Take a day to help others, and praise God for what He has blessed you with!

Day 8 "**Spring Cleaning**" - Take a day to go through your closet and get rid of anything that doesn't fit you anymore. If you haven't worn something in years, get rid of it. Donate these items to a local non-profit organization, and you will not only have a cleaner closet, but you will have a good mindset because you helped out someone in need. Do you have a little black dress that you want to fit into again? Hang it up and look at it for inspiration. Or go through your old pictures and organize them. Find an old picture of you at a time in your life where you were the happiest, and hang it on the refrigerator. It will help you stop and think before you grab that piece of cheesecake! Pray to the Lord for guidance and to give you strength!

Day 9 "**Positively Positive**" - An ugly personality will always ruin a beautiful face. Live your life with excess positivity. When you ooze positive energy, it rubs off on others. Everyone wants to be around someone who is happy. Negativity can be stressful and can hold you down, so learn to love yourself for who you are. Walk up to someone you would normally not talk to, and give them a compliment. Send a note or email to someone just expressing your sincere gratitude. Raise their spirits! Praise God for the joy in your life!

Day 10 "**Be Thankful**" - Make a list of things you are thankful for this month. Start with things like the air we breathe, the flowers, the sky, the mountains, the beach. Thank God for this wonderful world we live in. Then list everything from your toothbrush in the morning, to your coffee mug at the office, to your bed at night. Just sit for a minute and praise the Lord all the good in your life! Once you have that list, type it up, and use it to reflect each month on all the good things in your life!

Day 11 "**Gratitude Day**" - You worked hard today, and you earned it! Go treat yourself to a nice pedicure or manicure and lunch. And if you can't do this today, schedule an appointment for yourself, and *keep it*! This is also a good time to look at your calendar for the next month and make sure you have scheduled some "me-time" in the next few weeks. Remember that if you are tired and out-of-shape, you will not be working and thinking at your optimum performance. It's very important to take some time to yourself and treat yourself to some relaxation. Reflect on all the good things you have in life, and be grateful for what God has given you.

Day 12 "Moving On" - Toxic relationships drain your energy, affect your mood, and even can lower your self-esteem. Take an honest look at how you feel when you spend time with certain friends, co-workers, or family members. Ask yourself if they are holding you back or supporting you in being truly happy and fulfilled. If they are holding you back and are constantly saying "no" and "you can't do that," make the bold move to say "I can and I will!" Talk to this person with kindness and sincerity, and you will both be able to walk away with a smile. Praise God for giving you the ability to make your dreams happen!

Day 13 "Be Bold" - Do you want to talk to your boss about something that's been on your mind? Well, today is the day! Identify proactive ways to move towards your ultimate goal, whether it's asking your boss for a new assignment, taking courses that will expand your qualifications, or exploring new opportunities and business ideas. If you can go to work with a positive mindset and some new ways to help your career, you should see a new positive impact on your life. Praise the Lord for your job, and ask Him for guidance on how to be a better employee or boss.

Day 14 "Just Do It" - Today is the day to try something new. You only live once, so try something you never have before—something as simple as new food, or as crazy as going on an 80 ft roller coaster. Whatever your new thrill may be, find joy in the new memories and embrace them. You may not have the time today to go to a theme park or rock climb, but you can certainly find the time to schedule this! Even if it's registering for a 5k run that benefits a local cancer society, just do it! You will feel so great once you have fulfilled this goal! Praise God for giving you the freedom to do this!

Day 15 – "Clear the Clutter" - Clean out your car! We often use our car as another storage area, but clutter is clutter. Whether at home, in the car, or at your office, clutter and mess will affect your ability to think clearly and create positive flow. So take the time today to clean up your car and workspace. Clean out your junk drawer. It's time to get organized! People who are organized are more positive. And the more positive you are, the better your attitude is toward yourself and others. Your confidence will increase, and your fear will subside. Praise the Lord for all the little things in your life!

Day 16 "Meditate" - That's right, I said it! The word that most of us fear we can't do…that is, until we try it. Meditation is a real gift to yourself — it helps reduce stress, keep small irritations in perspective, and grounds you when you most need it. Just start small and focus on your breathing for five minutes at a time until you get the hang of it. Also, yoga is a great way to stay fit and healthy. Who wouldn't want to use a healthy way to find some serenity in this chaotic world? If you can't get to a Yoga class, find a quiet space for just you and God, and give thanks for the peace you have in your life!

Day 17 "Something New" - Make it a point to learn at least one new thing today. Research the name of a flower that grows in your garden, the capital of a far-off country, or even some new words in a different language. If you have children, spend some time with them today asking them to teach you something new. You'll be surprised to see how special your child feels that he has learned something his parent doesn't know. It's a win-win! If it's time for bed and you can't identify anything you've learned that day, take out your dictionary and learn a new word. Praise God for this ability!

Day 18 "No More Wasting Time" - Identify some ways in which you regularly waste time, and limit the time that you're going to spend on these activities each day. For example: watch no more than half an hour of television a day, or spend no more than half an hour each day on social media sites. By focusing on your own personal needs and not those that you see on TV or on Facebook, you will learn new things you didn't know about yourself. Use this extra time to do things that help you really feel better about yourself, or spend time with a family member. Whatever you do, spend this time praising God for these moments!

Day 19 "Eat Healthy" - Choose one food that constantly sabotages your efforts to eat healthier. Is it that decadent cheesecake from the bakery around the corner? Or that deep-dish pizza from your favorite Italian restaurant? Or your favorite potato chips? Just give it up. And find healthy foods that can replace these items. There are many desserts online made with yogurts and honey instead of creams and sugars. And they taste just as good! You just need to dedicate some time to making this change. Eating healthy is all about feeling good. Pray to God for the strength to eat healthier from this day forward!

Day 20 "Scrapbook" - Identify someone important in your life, and make that person a scrapbook. Gather pictures of all the things you and your loved one do together. Give this scrapbook (or one simple page of pictures) you created to the person you made it for. Making someone you love feel good about themselves will not only help their mood, but yours as well. Showing your love and admiration for others is such a great way to put a smile on your face. Even if you just send one picture in an email with a quick note thanking that person for her friendship, a little goes a long way. *Everyone* deserves to feel loved and special. Praise God for giving you such a wonderful person in your life!

Day 21 "Connections" - Today, connect with someone new. Greet a neighbor you've never spoken to before; follow someone new on Twitter (during your half hour of social media time!), or leave a comment on a new blog. Do something spontaneous. You never know what could happen when you talk to someone new. You could secure a new deal, find a new client, establish a new friendship, or even find the love of your life. Be courageous and brave and know that you were put on this earth to help others. Reach out. Pray for them, and see where God leads this new relationship!

Day 22 "Hugs for Everyone" - Give a few random hugs today. It may sound crazy and totally out of your comfort zone, but you need spontaneity. Hug an old lady, the person who makes your Starbucks drink, or that crazy neighbor. Someone could be having a horrible day and need a complete stranger to turn it all around. You will be surprised to see how quickly the recipient's mood changes. Giving someone affection could be the one thing that helps them to change their ways. Everyone has their dark moments, and we all could just use a hug sometimes! Praise the Lord for your happiness and the courage to help others find theirs!

Day 23 "Day of Praise" - Think long and hard about all the accomplishments you have achieved in your life. From giving birth, to winning a race, to reaching a goal at work—feel the joy and happiness you experienced during these times. Simply be thankful. Be thankful ALL DAY long! And make sure you offer thanks when anyone does anything for you! And don't just say a quick "thank you". Ask for the manager's card, and send a note thanking her for hiring such an awesome employee. Or get a colleague's personal address, and send a little note. Write one today! Praise God for all your accomplishments!

Day 24 "Best Day Ever" - Before bed, write down three good things that happened today. You may choose to use a journal or your computer to write about the events, but it is important that you have a physical record. Seeing the positivity of events, or even things you saw others do, can help you better yourself and motivate you to improve on your own life even more! Make this day the best day ever by actually creating the best day ever! You don't have to be on vacation or winning the lottery to have the best day ever. It's all mind-set. Give thanks to God for all that you have done and all that you will do!

Day 25 "Love Your Enemies" - Take a look at the relationships in your life. Are you having a difficult time getting along with someone? They may just have suffered the loss of a loved one or be in a difficult situation at home, so remember to show them love regardless. When someone is having a difficult time, kind words or actions may be all it takes to turn the relationship around. They may or may not change, but it's not up to you to change them! It's up to you to do good and feel good about yourself! Pray to the Lord for guidance to better help others!

Day 26 "A New Exercise" - Plan an organized exercise or yoga class. If possible, make it something you have never tried before—a Reiki session, or a Pilates class, or even a line dancing class. Just remember to make it something you enjoy. Keep an open mind, and consider choosing something you may have been avoiding. If you don't like it, try something else next month. If you like it, keep doing it. Do it over and over again, and soon enough you will be with a new group of friends who will hold you accountable for this new exercise program. Praise God for your strength!

Day 27 "Volunteer Day" - Look at a charity activity that interests you. You don't need to conquer the world. Every organization has small jobs that make a big difference. Charities need all the help they can get! Find a local cancer center or youth project that could use your help. Volunteer your time and efforts, and you will feel what it is like to give to others without expectation. It's an amazing feeling! Make a list of those you volunteer for, so you can help others if you wish. Pray to God to use you to help others!

Day 28 "Spa Day" - Plan a day of relaxation. Indulge in a much-needed facial or a nice massage. After all this work on your inner beauty, it may be time to step up and enhance that new glow you have about you from improving yourself. This may be something you choose to do by yourself or with a friend or loved one. This is all about relaxing, so make sure you choose your companion with careful consideration. The last thing you want to do is to get a pedicure and have to listen to someone complain about their spouse the whole time. You need to re-spect your soul enough to allow it to relax with pure positivity. Praise the Lord for your body, your temple.

Day 29 "Downtime" - Take a day and just do nothing. Unless you are working today, then don't do anything after work. Put your sweats on, and just read a book or magazine, or watch that movie that you have been waiting to see. This is a difficult task for most busy, driven people. But it's also very much needed! Order dinner instead of fixing a meal for the family. Have the kids buy lunch instead of making it. Leave the laundry until tomorrow. Give yourself a break, and just *relax*! Praise God for peace!

Day 30 "Celebrate You!" - Pull out your journal and write down all of your accomplishments from the last thirty days. Celebrate all of your positive improvements, and make a list of goals for the *next* thirty days!

Then, reward yourself with something that makes you feel wonderful. You deserve it! You are an amazing person, inside and out. You are worthy of all the good things in your life. You have many blessings in store for you. Have gratitude for where you have been, and be confident and courageous about your path ahead. Praise the Lord for helping you DETOX YOUR SOUL!

You can get this 30-day guide on your smart phone or tablet by simply searching for "Soul Detox" and downloading the app.

- For iTunes, the link is, https://itunes.apple.com/us/app/soul-detox/id733097087?mt=8.

- And for Google Play, the link is, https://play.google.com/store/apps/details?id=com.app_souldetox.layout&hl=en

It is a great way for you to help yourself stay focused on being positive. Having a positive mindset is what will help you continue to keep your soul detoxed. Having these daily thoughts and ideas with you at all times will help you with your life's goals. Just like anything you wish to be good at, change will take courage, consistency, and a coach. Let this book be yours. You can also schedule life coach sessions with me on my website: www.DetoxYourSoul.net. I will help you through your detox!

I know this may seem scary. You may have even skipped back to this part without even doing the hard work in the middle of this book. Just know that it's okay! We are all human, and we all have our struggles. Consider how many years it took me to rid my anger toward my biological father. I still get hurt feelings today, but I have now learned how to take those negative thoughts and create positive, uplifting ones. I get to choose my thoughts. I get to choose my responses. I get to choose my path. I am worth every bit of happiness in my life! You get to do all this as well! It's so exciting when we learn that we are in control of our own thoughts! Nobody can ever make us feel something we don't want to feel. Nobody. We are in control of our mind, body, and soul. I pray that God will soften your heart so that you are able to receive His grace and mercy that we all deserve. May God bless you and the lives of others you will touch along the way. He has big plans for you! Know that. Trust that. As you detox your soul, you will experience the love and happiness we were all made to receive. Enjoy every bit of it! It's absolutely amazing! YOU are incredible! YOU are worth it! YOU are loved! GOD BLESS YOU ALL!

www.ingramcontent.com/pod-product-compliance
Lightning Source LLC
Chambersburg PA
CBHW071219280526
45787CB00002B/728